Kidney Disease Recipes

Best Cookbook for Stopping Kidney Disease with Delicious and Easy Recipes. Start to Feel Better and Avoid Dialysis.

Robert Ashford

© Copyright 2021 - All rights reserved.

The content contained within this book may not be reproduced, duplicated or transmitted without direct written permission from the author or the publisher.

Under no circumstances will any blame or legal responsibility be held against the publisher, or author, for any damages, reparation, or monetary loss due to the information contained within this book. Either directly or indirectly.

Legal Notice:

This book is copyright protected. This book is only for personal use. You cannot amend, distribute, sell, use, quote or paraphrase any part, or the content within this book, without the consent of the author or publisher.

Disclaimer Notice:

Please note the information contained within this document is for educational and entertainment purposes only. All effort has been executed to present accurate, up to date, and reliable, complete information. No warranties of any kind are declared or implied. Readers acknowledge that the author is not engaging in the rendering of legal, financial, medical or professional advice. The content within this book has been derived from various sources. Please consult a licensed professional before attempting any techniques outlined in this book.

By reading this document, the reader agrees that under no circumstances is the author responsible for any losses, direct or indirect, which are incurred as a result of the use of information contained within this document, including, but not limited to, — errors, omissions, or inaccuracies.

Table of Contents

INTRODUCTION 6

Soups 7

   Mediterranean Vegetable Soup 7

   Steakhouse Soup 9

   Onion Soup 11

   Spaghetti Squash & Yellow Bell-Pepper Soup 13

Salads 15

   Thai Cucumber Salad 15

   Pear & Brie Salad 16

   Cucumber Salad 18

   Macaroni Salad 19

Kitchen Staples 20

   Homemade Mayonnaise 20

   Alfredo Sauce 21

   Cinnamon Applesauce 23

   Traditional Beef Stock 24

Lunch Recipes 26

   Appealing Green Salad 26

   Lunchtime Staple Sandwiches 28

   Healthier Pita Veggie Rolls 30

   Surprisingly Tasty Chicken Wraps 32

   Loveable Tortillas 33

Greek Style Pita Rolls 35

Energetic Fruity Salad 37

Delightful Pizza 39

Tastiest Meatballs 41

Dinner 43

Salmon with Spicy Honey 43

Turkey Sausages 45

Ground Turkey Burger 46

Stuffed Peppers 48

Pan Fried Beef and Broccoli 49

Rigatoni Spring Pasta 51

Seafood mains 53

Salmon & Pesto Salad 53

Cod & Green Bean Risotto 55

4-Ingredients Salmon Fillet 57

Poached Halibut in Orange Sauce 58

Oregano Salmon with Crunchy Crust 60

Cajun Catfish 61

Chili Mussels 62

Mackerel Skillet with Greens 64

Shrimp Paella 66

Fishen Papillote 68

Herby Chicken Stew 70

Monk-Fish Curry 72

Salmon Balls with Cream Cheese 74

Poultry and Meat mains 76

   Beef Brochettes 76

   Meat Loaf 78

   Chinese Beef Wraps 80

   Lamb with Zucchini & Couscous 82

   Grilled Skirt Steak 84

   Spiced Pork 86

   Spicy Lamb Curry 89

   Roast Beef 91

   Spiced Lamb Burgers 92

   Lemon & Herb Chicken Wraps 94

Vegetables mains 96

   Delicious Vegetarian Lasagne 96

   Mixed Pepper Paella 98

   Lentil Vegan Soup 100

   Thai Tofu Broth 102

   Chinese Tempeh Stir Fry 104

   Minted Zucchini Noodles 105

   Vegan Alfredo Fettuccine Pasta 107

INTRODUCTION

In the presence of disease, the kidneys lose their ability to filter out excess waste and minerals. It is important to set a diet with little protein and little sodium.

The first rule, experts recommend, to help patients with kidney failure especially when this is advanced, is to set a diet low in protein, sodium and phosphorus.

PROTEINS

It is necessary to reduce the amount of protein foods especially of animal origin (meat, fish, eggs, meats, cheeses and dairy products) and to a lesser extent of those rich in vegetable proteins (legumes), especially in main courses, including in the diet, where necessary, 'aproteinic' foods.

CALORIES

The caloric intake should be about 35 Kcal per kg (referred to the ideal weight of the person) per day in case of age under 60 years and 30 Kcal with age equal to or greater than 60 years. Below these values in the long term increases, in fact, the risk of malnutrition.

PHOSPHORUS

The values of this substance should be maintained within 8-10 mg/Kg body weight. In order to keep phosphorus values within the recommended range, it is important to limit and/or avoid cold cuts, dried legumes, dried fruit, chocolate, brewer's yeast, shrimps and offal, egg yolk, flour and bran, bitter cocoa powder.

SODIUM

Sodium is present in many foods and in large amounts. It is necessary to pay attention to table salt, avoid stock cubes, reduce the quantity and frequency of consumption of cold cuts and salami in general, foods in brine (capers, olives, canned meat and fish) and cheese.

Soups

Mediterranean Vegetable Soup

Preparation time:5 minutes
Cooking time:30 minutes
Servings:4

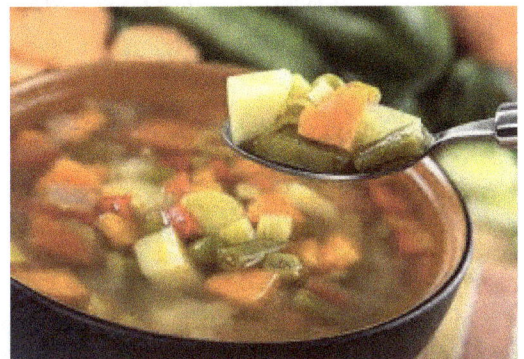

Ingredients:

- 1 tbsp. oregano
- 2 minced garlic cloves
- 1 tsp. black pepper
- 1 diced zucchini
- 1 cup diced eggplant
- 4 cups water
- 1 diced red pepper
- 1 tbsp. extra-virgin olive oil
- 1 diced red onion

Directions:

1. Soak the vegetables in warm water prior to use.
2. In a large pot, add the oil, chopped onion and minced garlic.
3. Sweat for 5 minutes on low heat.
4. Add the other vegetables to the onions and cook for 7-8 minutes.
5. Add the stock to the pan and bring to a boil on high heat.

6. Stir in the herbs, reduce the heat, and simmer for a further 20 minutes or until thoroughly cooked through.
7. Season with pepper to serve.

Nutrition:

- Calories 152
- Protein 1 g
- Carbs 6 g
- Fat 3 g
- Sodium (Na) 3 mg
- Potassium (K) 229 mg
- Phosphorus 45 mg

Steakhouse Soup

Preparation Time: 15 minutes
Cooking time:25 minutes
Servings:4

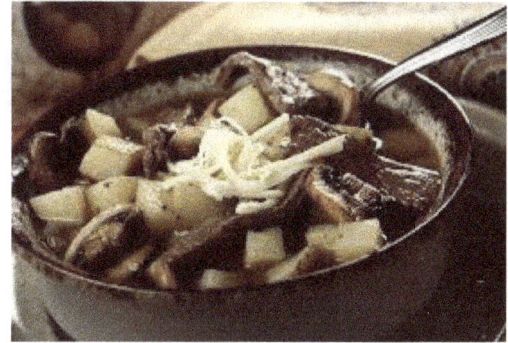

Ingredients:

- 2 tbsps. soy sauce
- 2 boneless and cubed chicken breasts.
- ¼ lb. halved and trimmed snow peas
- 1 tbsp. minced ginger root
- 1 minced garlic clove
- 1 cup water
- 2 chopped green onions
- 3 cups chicken stock
- 1 chopped carrot
- 3 sliced mushrooms

Directions:

1. Take a pot and combine ginger, water, chicken stock, Soy sauce (reduced salt) and garlic in this pot.
2. Let them boil on medium heat, mix in chicken pieces, and let them simmer on low heat for almost 15 minutes to tender chicken.
3. Stir in carrot and snow peas and simmer for almost 5 minutes.
4. Add mushrooms in this blend and continue cooking to tender vegetables for nearly 3 minutes.
5. Mix in the chopped onion and serve hot.

Nutrition:

- Calories 319
- Carbs 14g
- Fat 15g
- Potassium (K) 225 mg
- Protein 29g
- Sodium (Na) 389 mg
- Phosphorous 190

Onion Soup

Preparation time:15 minutes
Cooking time:45 minutes
Servings:6

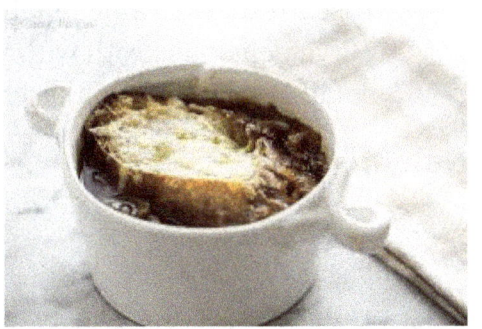

Ingredients:

- 2 tbsps. chicken stock
- 1 cup chopped Shiitake mushrooms
- 1 tbsp. minced chives
- 3 tsps. beef bouillon
- 1 tsp. grated ginger root
- ½ chopped carrot
- 1 cup sliced Portobello mushrooms
- 1 chopped onion
- ½ chopped celery stalk
- 2 quarts water
- ¼ tsp. minced garlic

Directions:

1. Take a saucepan and combine carrot, onion, celery, garlic, mushrooms (some mushrooms) and ginger in this pan. Add water, beef bouillon and chicken stock in this pan. Put this pot on high heat and let it boil. Decrease flame to medium and cover this pan to cook for almost 45 minutes.
2. Put all remaining mushrooms in one separate pot. Once the boiling mixture is completely done, put one strainer over this new bowl with mushrooms and

strain cooked soup in this pot over mushrooms. Discard solid-strained materials.
3. Serve delicious broth with yummy mushrooms in small bowls and sprinkle chives over each bowl.

Nutrition:

- Calories 22
- Fat 0g
- Sodium (Na) 602.3mg
- Potassium (K) 54.1mg
- Carbs 4.9g
- Protein 0.6g
- Phosphorus 15.8mg

Spaghetti Squash & Yellow Bell-Pepper Soup

Preparation time: 10 minutes
Cooking time: 45 minutes
Servings: 4

Ingredients:

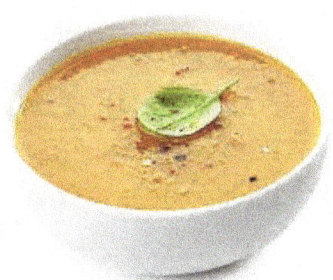

- 2 diced yellow bell peppers
- 2 chopped large garlic cloves
- 1 peeled and cubed spaghetti squash
- 1 quartered and sliced onion
- 1 tbsp. dried thyme
- 1 tbsp. coconut oil
- 1 tsp. curry powder
- 4 cups water

Directions:

1. Heat the oil in a large pan over medium-high heat before sweating the onions and garlic for 3-4 minutes.
2. Sprinkle over the curry powder.
3. Add the stock and bring to a boil over a high heat before adding the squash, pepper and thyme.
4. Turn down the heat, cover and allow to simmer for 25-30 minutes.
5. Continue to simmer until squash is soft if needed.
6. Allow to cool before blitzing in a blender/food processor until smooth.
7. Serve!

Nutrition:

- Calories 103
- Protein 2 g
- Carbs 17 g
- Fat 4 g
- Sodium (Na) 32 mg
- Potassium (K) 365 mg
- Phosphorus 50 mg

Salads

Thai Cucumber Salad

Preparation time:5 minutes
Cooking time:5 minutes
Servings:2

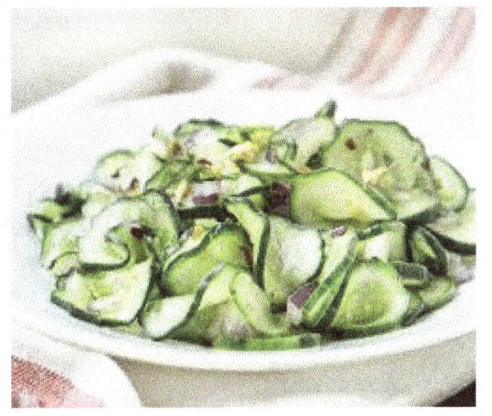

Ingredients:

- ¼ cup chopped peanuts
- ¼ cup white sugar
- ½ cup cilantro
- ¼ cup rice wine vinegar
- 3 cucumbers
- 2 jalapeno peppers

Directions:

1. In a bowl add all ingredients and mix well
2. Serve with dressing

Nutrition:

- Calories 20
- Fat 0g
- Sodium (Na) 85mg
- Carbs 5g
- Protein 1g
- Potassium (K) 190.4 mg
- Phosphorus 46.8mg

Pear & Brie Salad

Preparation time: 5 minutes
Cooking time: 0 minutes
Servings: 4

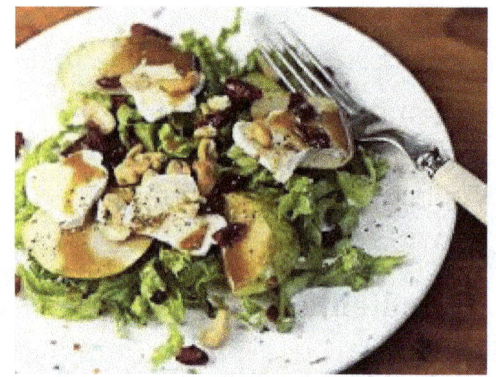

Ingredients:

- 1 tbsp. olive oil
- 1 cup arugula
- ½ lemon
- ½ cup canned pears
- ¼ cucumber
- ¼ cup chopped brie

Directions:

1. Peel and dice the cucumber.
2. Dice the pear.
3. Wash the arugula.
4. Combine salad in a serving bowl and crumble the brie over the top.
5. Whisk the olive oil and lemon juice together.
6. Drizzle over the salad.
7. Season with a little black pepper to taste and serve immediately.

Nutrition:

- Calories 54
- Protein 1 g
- Carbs 12 g
- Fat 7 g
- Sodium (Na) 57mg

- Potassium (K) 115 mg
- Phosphorus 67 mg

Cucumber Salad

Preparation time: 5 minutes
Cooking time: 5 minutes
Servings: 4

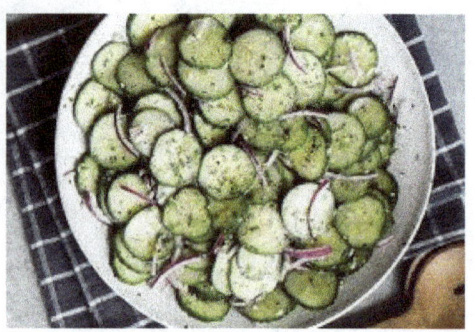

Ingredients:

- 1 tbsp. dried dill
- 1 onion
- ¼ cup water
- 1 cup vinegar
- 3 cucumbers
- ¾ cup white sugar

Directions:

1. In a bowl add all ingredients and mix well
2. Serve with dressing

Nutrition:

- Calories 49
- Fat 0.1g
- Sodium (Na) 341mg
- Potassium (K) 171mg
- Protein 0.8g
- Carbs 11g
- Phosphorus 24 mg

Macaroni Salad

Preparation time:5 minutes
Cooking time:5 minutes
Servings:4

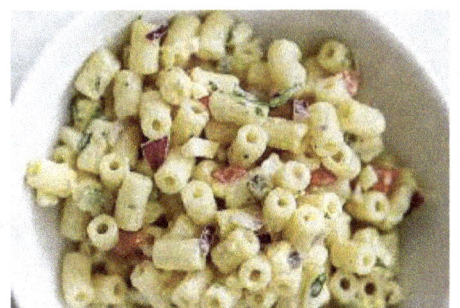

Ingredients:

- ¼ tsp. celery seed
- 2 hard-boiled eggs
- 2 cups salad dressing
- 1 onion
- 2 tsps. white vinegar
- 2 stalks celery
- 2 cups cooked macaroni
- 1 red bell pepper
- 2 tbsps. mustard

Directions:

1. In a bowl add all ingredients and mix well
2. Serve with dressing

Nutrition:

- Calories 360
- Fat 21g
- Sodium (Na) 400mg
- Carbs 36g
- Protein 6g
- Potassium (K) 68mg
- Phosphorus 36 mg

Kitchen Staples

Homemade Mayonnaise

Preparation Time: 5 minutes
Servings: 1 cup (1 tbsp = 1 serving)

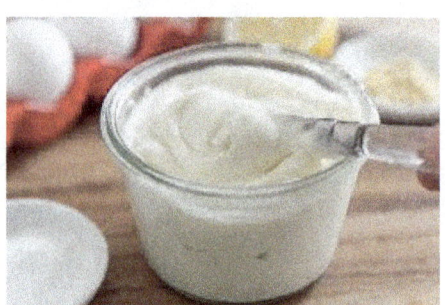

Ingredients:

- Egg yolks - 2
- Lemon juice – 1 ½ tsp
- Mustard powder – ¼ tsp
- Olive oil – ¾ cup

Directions:

1. In a bowl, whisk together the lemon juice, yolks, and mustard for 30 seconds or until well blended.
2. Add the olive oil in a thin, steady stream while whisking for 3 minutes or until the oil is emulsified and the mayonnaise is thick.
3. Store in the refrigerator.

Nutrition:

- Calories 97
- Fat 11g
- Carb 0g
- Phosphorus 9mg
- Potassium 3mg
- Sodium 1mg
- Protein 0g

Alfredo Sauce

Preparation Time: 10 minutes
Cooking Time: 10 minutes
Servings: ¼ cup, 8 servings

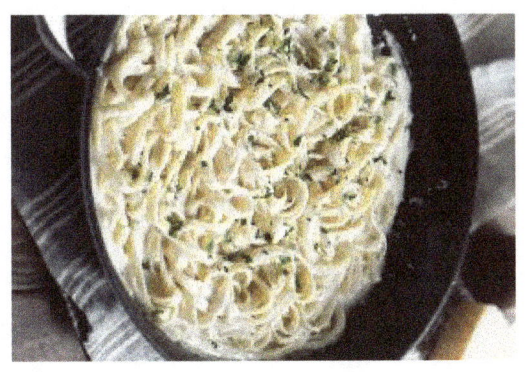

Ingredients:

- Unsalted butter – 2 tbsp
- All-purpose flour – 1 ½ tbsp.
- Minced garlic – 1 tsp
- Plain unsweetened rice milk - 1 cup
- Plain cream cheese – ¾ cup
- Parmesan cheese – 2 tbsp
- Ground nutmeg – ¼ tsp
- Ground black pepper, for seasoning

Directions:

1. Melt the butter in a saucepan.
2. Whisk in the flour and garlic to form a paste and continue whisking for 2 minutes to cook the flour.
3. Whisk in the rice milk and continue whisking for about 4 minutes or until the mixture is almost boiling and thick.
4. Whisk in the cream cheese, parmesan cheese, and nutmeg for 1 minute or until the sauce is smooth.
5. Remove the sauce from the heat and season with pepper.
6. Serve immediately over pasta.

Nutrition:

- Calories 98
- Fat 7g
- Carb 6g
- Phosphorus 66mg
- Potassium 70mg
- Sodium 141mg
- Protein 3g

Cinnamon Applesauce

Preparation Time: 10 minutes
Cooking Time: 30 minutes
Servings: 3 cups

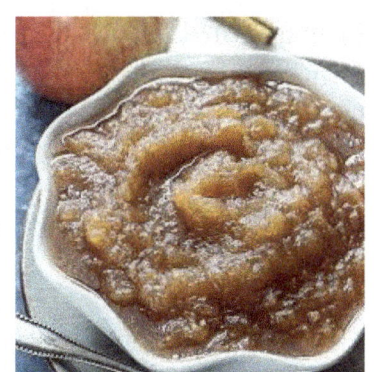

Ingredients:

- Apples – 8, peeled and sliced thin
- Water – ½ cup
- Ground cinnamon – 1 tsp
- Ground nutmeg – ¼ tsp
- Pinch ground allspice

Directions:

1. In a saucepan, put the water, apples, cinnamon, nutmeg, and allspice over medium heat.
2. Heat the apple mixture, frequently stirring, for 25 to 30 minutes or until the apples soften.
3. Remove the saucepan from the heat and mash the potatoes.
4. Let the applesauce cool.
5. Store in the refrigerator.

Nutrition:

- Calories 106
- Fat 0g
- Carb 28g
- Phosphorus 24mg
- Potassium 196mg
- Sodium 0mg
- Protein 1g

Traditional Beef Stock

Preparation Time: 15 minutes
Cooking Time: 13 hours
Servings: 8 cups

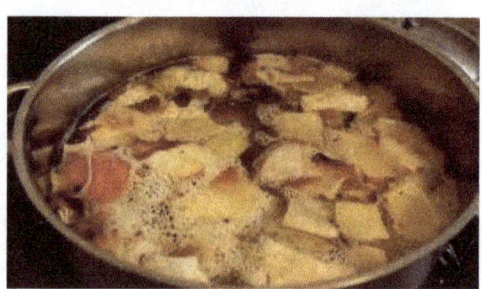

Ingredients:

- Beef marrow, knucklebones, or ribs – 2 pounds
- Celery stalk – 1, chopped
- Carrot – 1, peeled and chopped
- Sweet onion – ½, quartered
- Garlic – 3 cloves, crushed
- Black peppercorns - 1 tsp
- Thyme – 3 sprigs
- Bay leaves – 2
- Water

Directions:

1. Preheat the oven to 350F.
2. Place the bones in a deep baking pan and roast them in the oven for 30 minutes, turning once.
3. Transfer the roasted bones to a large stockpot and add the celery, carrots, onion, garlic, peppercorns, thyme, bay leaves, and enough water to cover the bones by about 3 inches.
4. Reduce the heat to low and simmer the stock for at least 12 hours. Check the broth every hour for the first 4 hours to skim off any foam from the top.
5. Remove from the heat and cool for 30 minutes.

6. Remove the large bones with tongs, and then strain the stock.
7. Store and use.

Nutrition: Facts Per Serving (1 cup serving)

- Calories 121
- Fat 5g
- Carb 2g
- Phosphorus 21mg
- Potassium 79mg
- Sodium 87mg
- Protein 4g

Lunch Recipes

Appealing Green Salad

Preparation Time: 50 minutes
Cooking Time: 15 minutes (4 servings, serving: 1 salad plate)

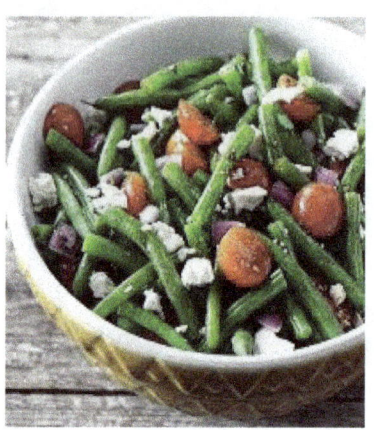

Ingredients:

- For Dressing:
  - 1 tbsp. of shallot, minced
  - 1/3 cup of olive oil
  - 2 tbsp. of fresh lemon juice
  - 1 tsp. of honey
  - Freshly ground black pepper, to taste
- For Salad:
  - 1½ cups of chopped broccoli florets
  - 1½ cups of shredded cabbage
  - 4 cups of chopped lettuce

Directions:

1. In a bowl, add all dressing ingredients and beat until well combined. Keep aside.
2. In another large bowl, mix all salad ingredients.
3. Add dressing and gently, toss to coat well.
4. Serve immediately.

Nutrition: Per Serving

- Calories 179
- Fat 17.1g

- Carbs 7.5g
- Protein 1.7g
- Fiber 1.9g
- Potassium 249mg
- Sodium 21mg

Lunchtime Staple Sandwiches

Preparation Time: 40 minutes
Cooking Time: 15 minutes
(2 servings, serving: ½ sandwich)

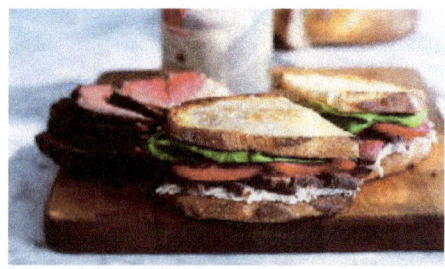

Ingredients:

- 3 tsp. of low-sodium mayonnaise
- 2 toasted white bread slices
- 3 tbsp. of chopped unsalted cooked turkey
- 2 thin apple slices
- 2 tbsp. of low-fat cheddar cheese
- 1 tsp. of olive oil

Directions:

1. Spread mayonnaise over each slice evenly.
2. Place turkey over 1 slice, followed by apple slices and cheese.
3. Cover with remaining slice to make sandwich.
4. Grease a large nonstick frying pan with oil and heat on medium heat.
5. Place the sandwich in frying pan and with the back of spoon, gently, press down.
6. Cook for about 1-2 minutes.
7. Carefully, flip the whole sandwich and cook for about 1-2 minutes.
8. Transfer the sandwich into serving plate.
9. With a knife, carefully cut the sandwich diagonally ad serve.

Nutrition: Per Serving

- Calories 239
- Fat 8.5g
- Carbs 37.2g
- Protein 7g
- Fiber 5.6g
- Potassium 294mg
- Sodium 169mg

Healthier Pita Veggie Rolls

Preparation Time: 30 minutes
Cooking Time: 15 minutes (6 servings, serving: ½ roll)

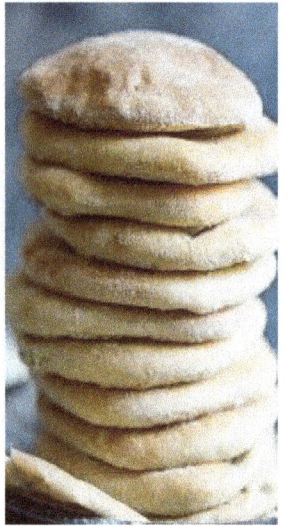

Ingredients:

- 1 cup of shredded romaine lettuce
- 1 seeded and chopped red bell pepper
- ½ cup of chopped cucumber
- 1 small seeded and chopped tomato
- 1 small chopped red onion
- 1 finely minced garlic clove
- 1 tbsp. of olive oil
- ½ tbsp. of fresh lemon juice
- Freshly ground black pepper, to taste
- 3 (6½-inch) pita breads

Directions:

1. In a large bowl, add all ingredients except pita breads and gently toss to coat well.
2. Arrange pita breads onto serving plates.
3. Place veggie mixture in the center of each pita bread evenly. Roll the pita bread and serve.

Nutrition Per Serving

- Calories 120
- Fat 2.8g
- Carbs 20.7g

- Protein 3.3g
- Fiber 1.5g
- Potassium 156mg
- Sodium 164mg

Surprisingly Tasty Chicken Wraps

Preparation Time: 50 minutes
Cooking Time: 15 minutes (4 servings, serving: 1 wrap)

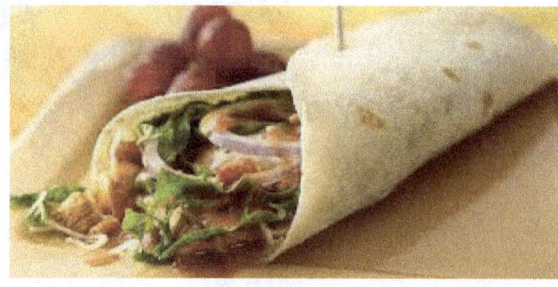

Ingredients:

- 4-ounce of cut into strips unsalted cooked chicken breast
- ½ cup of hulled and thinly sliced fresh strawberries
- 1 thinly sliced English cucumber
- 1 tbsp. of chopped fresh mint leaves
- 4 large lettuce leaves

Directions:

1. In a large bowl, add all ingredients except lettuce leaves and gently toss to coat well.
2. Place the lettuce leaves onto serving plates.
3. Divide the chicken mixture over each leaf evenly.
4. Serve immediately.

Nutrition Per Serving

- Calories 74
- Fat 2.3g
- Carbs 4.7g
- Protein 8.9g
- Fiber 0.9g
- Potassium 235mg
- Sodium 27mg

Loveable Tortillas

Preparation Time: 60 minutes
Cooking Time: 15 minutes (8 servings, serving: ½ tortilla)

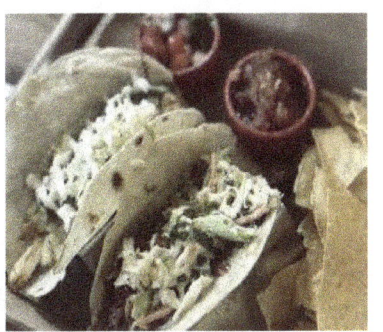

Ingredients:

- ½ cup of low-sodium mayonnaise
- 1 finely minced small garlic clove
- 8-ounce of chopped unsalted cooked chicken
- ½ of seeded and chopped red bell pepper
- ½ of seeded and chopped green bell pepper
- 1 chopped red onion
- 4 (6-ounce) warmed corn tortillas

Directions:

1. In a bowl, mix mayonnaise and garlic.
2. In another bowl, mix chicken and vegetables.
3. Arrange the tortillas onto smooth surface.
4. Spread mayonnaise mixture over each tortilla evenly.
5. Place chicken mixture over ¼ of each tortilla.
6. Fold the outside edges inward and roll up like a burrito.
7. Secure each tortilla with toothpicks to secure the filling.
8. Cut each tortilla in half and serve.

Nutrition Per Serving

- Calories 296
- Fat 8.2g

- Carbs 44g
- Protein 13.5g
- Fiber 5.9g
- Potassium 262mg
- Sodium 162mg

Greek Style Pita Rolls

Preparation Time: 20 minutes
Cooking Time: 15 minutes (4 servings, serving: ½ roll)

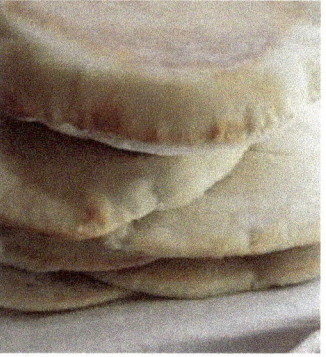

Ingredients:

- 2 (6½-inch) pita breads
- 1 tbsp. of low-fat cream cheese
- 1 peeled, cored and thinly sliced apple
- Olive oil cooking spray, as required
- 1/8 tsp. of ground cinnamon

Directions:

1. Preheat the oven to 400 degrees F.
2. In a microwave safe plate, place tortillas and microwave for about 10 seconds to soften.
3. Spread the cream cheese over each tortilla evenly.
4. Arrange apple slices in the center of each tortilla evenly.
5. Roll tortillas to secure the filling.
6. Arrange the tortilla rolls onto a baking sheet in a single layer.
7. Spray the rolls with cooking spray evenly and sprinkle with cinnamon.
8. Bake for about 10 minutes or until top becomes golden brown.

Nutrition Per Serving

- Calories 129
- Fat 2.2g
- Carbs 24.6g
- Protein 3.3g
- Fiber 2.1g
- Potassium 102mg
- Sodium 176mg

Energetic Fruity Salad

Preparation Time: 20 minutes
Cooking Time: 15 minutes (12 servings, serving: 1 salad plate)

Ingredients:

- For Dressing:
    - ½ cup of fresh pineapple juice
    - 2 tbsp. of fresh lemon juice
- For Salad:
    - 2 cups of hulled and sliced fresh strawberries
    - 2 cups of fresh blackberries
    - 2 cups of fresh blueberries
    - 1 cup of halved seedless red grapes
    - 1 cup of halved seedless red grapes
    - 6 cored and chopped fresh apples

Directions:

1. In a bowl, add all dressing ingredients and beat until well combined. Keep aside.
2. In another large bowl, mix all salad ingredients.
3. Add dressing and gently, toss to coat well.
4. Refrigerate, covered to chill before serving.

Nutrition Per Serving

- Calories 116
- Fat 0.5g
- Carbs 29.3g
- Protein 1.2g

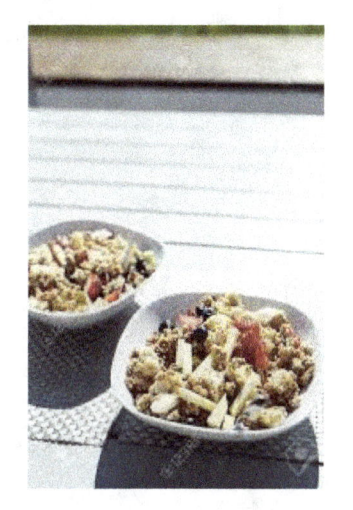

- Fiber 5.3g
- Potassium 276mg
- Sodium 3mg

Delightful Pizza

Preparation Time: 40 minutes
Cooking Time: 15 minutes (4 servings, serving: ½ pizza)

Ingredients:

- 2 (6½-inch) pita breads
- 3 tbsp. of low-sodium tomato sauce
- 3-ounce of cubed unsalted cooked chicken
- ¼ cup of chopped onion
- 2 tbsp. of crumbled feta cheese

Directions:

1. Preheat the oven to 350 degrees F. Grease a baking sheet.
2. Arrange the pita breads onto prepared baking sheet.
3. Spread the barbecue sauce over each pita bread evenly.
4. Top with chicken and onion evenly and sprinkle with cheese.
5. Bake for about 11-13 minutes.
6. Cut each pizza in half and serve.

Nutrition Per Serving

- Calories 133
- Fat 2g
- Carbs 18.2g
- Protein 9.8g

- Fiber 1g
- Potassium 0mg
- Sodium 287mg

Tastiest Meatballs

Preparation Time: 10 minutes
Cooking Time: 15 minutes
(6 servings, serving: 3-4 meatballs with ½ cup lettuce)

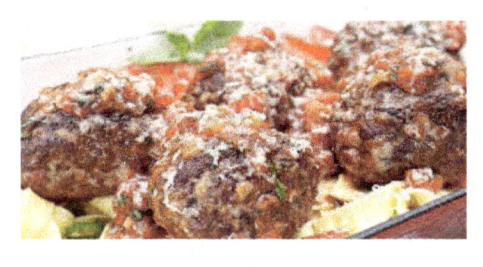

Ingredients:

- 1 pound of lean ground chicken
- 1 tbsp. of olive oil
- 1 tsp. of minced garlic
- 2 tbsp. of minced fresh cilantro
- ½ tsp. of ground cumin
- ½ tsp. of crushed red pepper flakes
- 3 cups of torn lettuce leaves

Directions:

1. Preheat the oven to 400 degrees F.
2. Line a large baking sheet with parchment paper.
3. For meatballs in a large bowl, add all ingredients and mix until well combined.
4. Make desired sized balls from mixture.
5. Arrange the meatballs into prepared baking sheet in a single layer.
6. Bake for about 15-20 minutes or till done completely.
7. Divide lettuce in serving plates evenly. Top with meatballs and serve.

Nutrition Per Serving

- Calories 126

- Fat 6.5 g
- Carbs 1.2g
- Protein 15.5g
- Fiber 0.5g
- Potassium 49mg
- Sodium 85mg

Dinner

Salmon with Spicy Honey

Servings: 2

Preparation Time: 15 Minutes

Ingredients:

- 16 oz. salmon fillet
- 3 tbsp. honey
- 3/4 tsp. lemon peel
- 3 bowls arugula salad
- 1/2 tsp. black pepper
- 1/2 tsp. garlic powder
- 2 tsp. olive oil
- 1 tsp. hot water

Directions:

1. Prepare a small bowl with some hot water and put in honey, grated lemon peel, ground pepper, and garlic powder.
2. Spread the mixture over salmon fillets.
3. Warm some olive oil at a medium heat and add spiced salmon fillet and cook for 4 minutes.
4. Turn the fillets on one side then on the other side.
5. Continue to cook for other 4 minutes at a reduced heat and try to check when the salmon fillets flake easily.

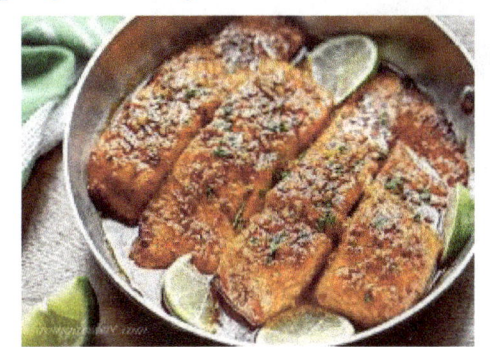

6. Put some arugula on each plate and add the salmon fillets on top, adding some aromatic herbs or some dill. Serve and enjoy!

Nutrition:

- Calories 320
- Protein 23 g
- Sodium 65 mg
- Potassium 450 mg
- Phosphorus 250 mg

Turkey Sausages

Servings: 2

Preparation Time: 10 Minutes

Ingredients:

- 1/4 tsp. salt
- 1/8 tsp. garlic powder
- 1/8 tsp. onion powder
- 1 tsp. fennel seed
- 1 pound 7% fat ground turkey

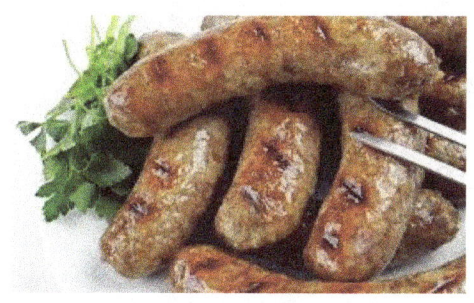

Directions:

1. Press the fennel seed and in a small cup put together turkey with fennel seed, garlic and onion powder and salt.
2. Cover the bowl and refrigerate overnight.
3. Prepare the turkey with seasoning into different portions with a circle form and press them into patties ready to be cooked.
4. Cook at a medium heat until browned.
5. Cook it for 1 to 2 minutes per side and serve them hot. Enjoy!

Nutrition:

- Calories 55
- Protein 7 g
- Sodium 70 mg
- Potassium 105 mg
- Phosphorus 75 mg

Ground Turkey Burger

Servings: 2

Preparation Time: 15 Minutes

Ingredients:

- 1 pound ground lean turkey
- 6 hamburger buns
- 1/2 dish red onion
- 1/2 dish green bell pepper
- 1/2 spoon chicken grilled blend seasoning
- 2 tsp. brown sugar
- 1 tbsp. Worcestershire sauce
- 1 cup low sodium tomato sauce

Directions:

1. Cook the turkey at medium heat.
2. Cut little pieces of onion and green bell pepper.
3. Mix the sauce, the grilled blend seasoning and tomato sauce.
4. Add seasoning to the turkey mixture and cook for 10 minutes.
5. Prepare 5 portions and put in burger buns. Serve and enjoy!

Nutrition:

- Calories 28
- Protein 24 g
- Sodium 285 mg

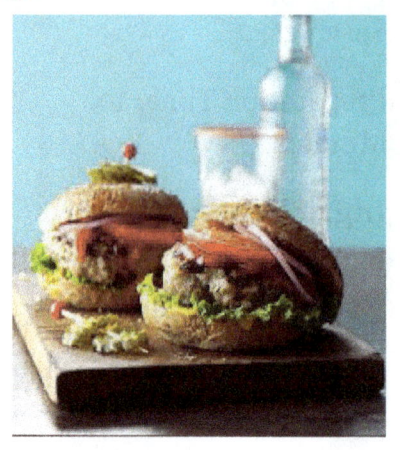

- Potassium 510 mg
- Phosphorus 235 mg

Stuffed Peppers

Servings: 2

Preparation Time: 1 Hour 15 Minutes

Ingredients:

- 4 bell peppers
- 1 tbsp. dried parsley
- 2 cups cooked white rice
- 2 tsp. garlic powder
- 1 tsp. black pepper
- 3/4 pound ground beef
- 1/2 bowl chopped onion
- 3 oz. unsalted tomato sauce

Directions:

1. Remove the seeds from black peppers
2. Preheat the oven at 375°F (or 200°C)
3. Roast the beef and add onion, rice, parsley, black pepper, garlic powder and tomato sauce to the beef.
4. Boil slowly for 10 minutes.
5. Feel the bell peppers with mixture and bake in the oven for one hour. Serve and enjoy!

Nutrition:

- Calories 260
- Protein 20 g
- Sodium 210 mg
- Potassium 550 mg
- Phosphorus 208 mg

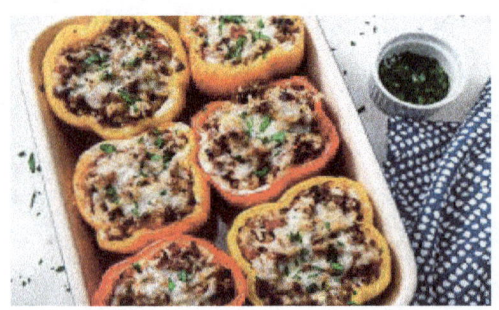

Pan Fried Beef and Broccoli

Servings: 2

Preparation Time: 25 Minutes

Ingredients:

- 2 garlic small slices
- 1 tomato
- 8 oz. uncooked lean sirloin beef
- 12 oz. frozen broccoli stir fry vegetable blend
- 2 little spoons peanut oil
- 1/4 cup low sodium chicken consommé
- 1 tsp. cornstarch
- 2 tsp. low sodium soy sauce
- 2 bowls cooked rice

Directions:

1. Cut the garlic cloves and tomato.
2. Cut the beef into strips and place the broccoli in the microwave for 3-4 minutes.
3. In a wok pan heat oil and the garlic to make them fragrant. Add vegetable blend cooking it for about 4 minutes or more and remove from pan.
4. Add the beef in the same pot and cook it for around 7-8 minutes, then prepare the sauce putting together the consommé, the soy sauce and cornstarch.
5. Add vegetables, sauce, tomato and heat them with the beef until the sauce is ready.
6. Serve the dish with brown rice. Enjoy!

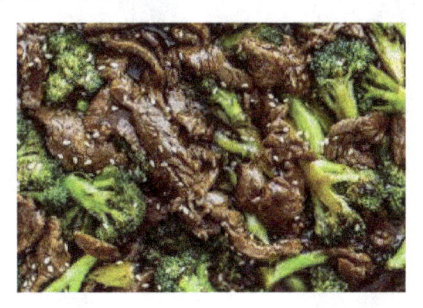

Nutrition:

- Calories 370
- Protein 18 g
- Sodium 350 mg
- Potassium 550 mg
- Phosphorus 250 mg

Rigatoni Spring Pasta

Servings: 2

Preparation Time: 20 Minutes

Ingredients:

- 12 oz. rigatoni pasta (you can also use fusilli or farfalle pasta)
- 12 oz. vegetables (carrots, broccoli and zucchini or any other fresh vegetable)
- 2 portions half and half creamer
- Grated parmesan cheese

Directions:

1. Boil the water and when the water starts producing bubbles, put the pasta in it. For Rigatoni it will take around 11 minutes to cook. In the meantime, put the cut and diced vegetables into a pan with some olive oil in it. Mix the vegetables until they are soft and ready, adding the two small portions of half and half creamer.
2. When the pasta boils, drain it in a strainer and put it in the pan where you have prepared the vegetables.
3. Mix everything together and put the pasta on a dish, adding some parmesan cheese on top. (If you prefer you can add the parmesan cheese when you are mixing the ingredients in the pan at a medium heat).
4. Then serve hot. Enjoy!

Nutrition:

- Calories 253
- Protein 10 g
- Sodium 115 mg
- Potassium 250 mg
- Phosphorus 153 mg

Seafood mains

Salmon & Pesto Salad

Preparation time:5 minutes
Cooking time:15 minutes
Servings:2

Ingredients:

- ➢ For the pesto:
    - 1 minced garlic clove
    - ½ cup fresh arugula
    - ¼ cup extra virgin olive oil
    - ½ cup fresh basil
    - 1 tsp. black pepper
- ➢ For the salmon:
    - 4 oz. skinless salmon fillet
    - 1 tbsp. coconut oil
- ➢ For the salad:
    - ½ juiced lemon
    - 2 sliced radishes
    - ½ cup iceberg lettuce
    - 1 tsp. black pepper

Directions:

1. Prepare the pesto by blending all the ingredients for the pesto in a food processor or by grinding with a pestle and mortar. Set aside.
2. Add a skillet to the stove on medium-high heat and melt the coconut oil.
3. Add the salmon to the pan.

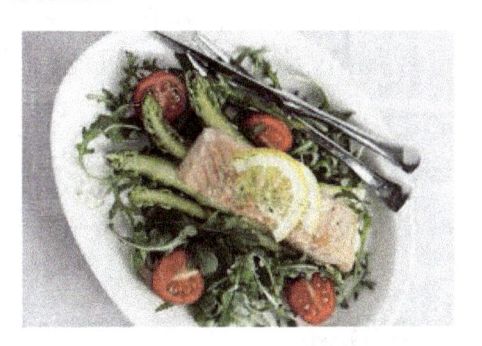

4. Cook for 7-8 minutes and turn over.
5. Cook for a further 3-4 minutes or until cooked through.
6. Remove fillets from the skillet and allow to rest.
7. Mix the lettuce and the radishes and squeeze over the juice of ½ lemon.
8. Flake the salmon with a fork and mix through the salad.
9. Toss to coat and sprinkle with a little black pepper to serve.

Nutrition:

- Calories 221
- Protein 13 g
- Carbs 1 g
- Fat 34 g
- Sodium (Na) 80 mg
- Potassium (K) 119 mg
- Phosphorus 158 mg

Cod & Green Bean Risotto

Preparation time: 4 minutes
Cooking time: 40 minutes
Servings: 2

Ingredients:

- ½ cup arugula
- 1 finely diced white onion
- 4 oz. cod fillet
- 1 cup white rice
- 2 lemon wedges
- 1 cup boiling water
- ¼ tsp. black pepper
- 1 cup low sodium chicken broth
- 1 tbsp. extra virgin olive oil
- ½ cup green beans

Directions:

1. Heat the oil in a large pan on medium heat.
2. Sauté the chopped onion for 5 minutes until soft before adding in the rice and stirring for 1-2 minutes.
3. Combine the broth with boiling water.
4. Add half of the liquid to the pan and stir slowly.
5. Slowly add the rest of the liquid whilst continuously stirring for up to 20-30 minutes.
6. Stir in the green beans to the risotto.
7. Place the fish on top of the rice, cover and steam for 10 minutes.

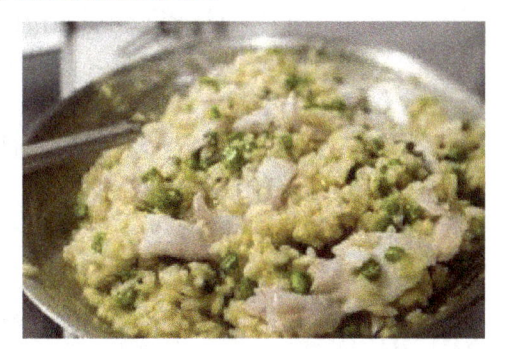

8. Ensure the water does not dry out and keep topping up until the rice is cooked thoroughly.
9. Use your fork to break up the fish fillets and stir into the rice.
10. Sprinkle with freshly ground pepper to serve and a squeeze of fresh lemon.
11. Garnish with the lemon wedges and serve with the arugula.

Nutrition:

- Calories 221
- Protein 12 g
- Carbs 29 g
- Fat 8 g
- Sodium (Na) 398 mg
- Potassium (K) 347 mg
- Phosphorus 241 mg

4-Ingredients Salmon Fillet

Preparation Time: 5 minutes

Cooking Time: 25 minutes

Servings: 1

Ingredients:

- 4 oz salmon fillet
- ½ teaspoon salt
- 1 teaspoon sesame oil
- ½ teaspoon sage

Directions:

1. Rub the fillet with salt and sage.
2. Place the fish in the tray and sprinkle it with sesame oil.
3. Cook the fish for 25 minutes at 365F.
4. Flip the fish carefully onto another side after 12 minutes of cooking.

Nutrition:

- Calories 191
- Fat 11.6
- Fiber 0.1
- Carbs 0.2
- Protein 22

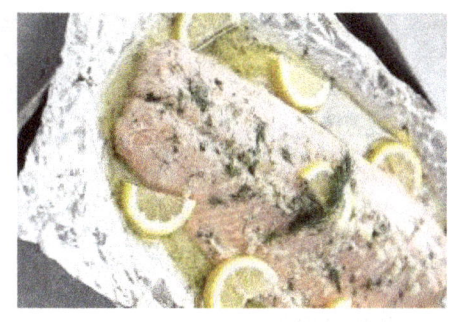

Poached Halibut in Orange Sauce

Preparation Time: 10 minutes

Cooking Time: 10 minutes

Servings: 4

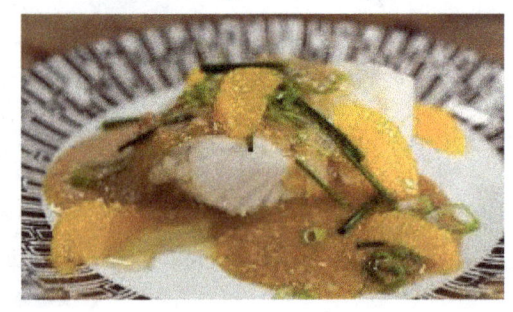

Ingredients:

- 1-pound halibut
- 1/3 cup butter
- 1 rosemary sprig
- ½ teaspoon ground black pepper
- 1 teaspoon salt
- 1 teaspoon honey
- ¼ cup of orange juice
- 1 teaspoon cornstarch

Directions:

1. Put butter in the saucepan and melt it.
2. Add rosemary sprig.
3. Sprinkle the halibut with salt and ground black pepper.
4. Put the fish in the boiling butter and poach it for 4 minutes.
5. Meanwhile, pour orange juice in the skillet. Add honey and bring the liquid to boil.
6. Add cornstarch and whisk until the liquid will start to be thick.
7. Then remove it from the heat.

8. Transfer the poached halibut in the plate and cut it on 4.
9. Place every fish serving in the serving plate and top with orange sauce.

Nutrition:

- Calories 349
- Fat 29.3
- Fiber 0.1
- Carbs 3.2
- Protein 17.8

Oregano Salmon with Crunchy Crust

Preparation Time: 10 minutes

Cooking Time: 2 hours

Servings: 2

Ingredients:

- 8 oz salmon fillet
- 2 tablespoons panko breadcrumbs
- 1 oz Parmesan, grated
- 1 teaspoon dried oregano
- 1 teaspoon sunflower oil

Directions:

1. In the mixing bowl combine together panko breadcrumbs, Parmesan, and dried oregano.
2. Sprinkle the salmon with olive oil and coat in the breadcrumb's mixture.
3. After this, line the baking tray with baking paper.
4. Place the salmon in the tray and transfer in the preheated to the 385F oven.
5. Bake the salmon for 25 minutes.

Nutrition:

- Calories 245
- Fat 12.8
- Fiber 0.6
- Carbs 5.9
- Protein 27.5

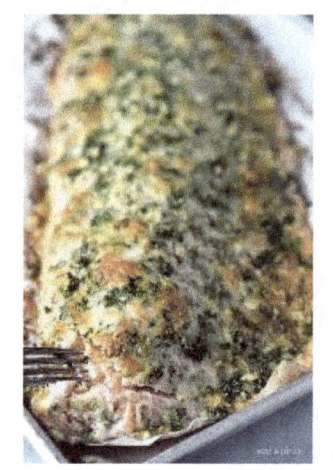

Cajun Catfish

Preparation Time: 10 minutes

Cooking Time: 10 minutes

Servings: 4

Ingredients:

1. 16 oz catfish steaks (4 oz each fish steak)
2. 1 tablespoon cajun spices
3. 1 egg, beaten
4. 1 tablespoon sunflower oil
5. Directions:
6. Pour sunflower oil in the skillet and preheat it until shimmering.
7. Meanwhile, dip every catfish steak in the beaten egg and coat in Cajun spices.
8. Place the fish steaks in the hot oil and roast them for 4 minutes from each side.
9. The cooked catfish steaks should have a light brown crust.

Nutrition:

- Calories 263
- Fat 16.7
- Fiber 0
- Carbs 0.1
- Protein 26.3

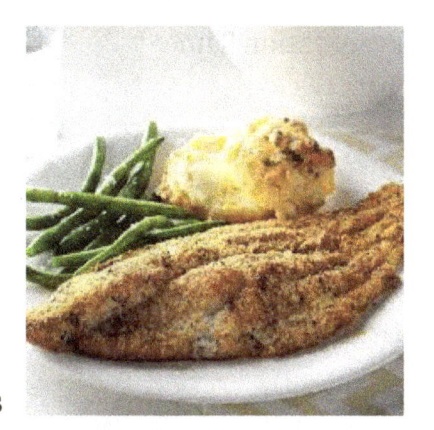

Chili Mussels

Preparation Time: 7 minutes

Cooking Time: 10 minutes

Servings: 4

Ingredients:

- 1-pound mussels
- 1 chili pepper, chopped
- 1 cup chicken stock
- ½ cup milk
- 1 teaspoon olive oil
- 1 teaspoon minced garlic
- 1 teaspoon ground coriander
- ½ teaspoon salt
- 1 cup fresh parsley, chopped
- 4 tablespoons lemon juice

Directions:

1. Pour milk in the saucepan.
2. Add chili pepper, chicken stock, olive oil, minced garlic, ground coriander, salt, and lemon juice.
3. Bring the liquid to boil and add mussels.
4. Boil the mussel for 4 minutes or until they will open shells.
5. Then add chopped parsley and mix up the meal well.
6. Remove it from the heat.

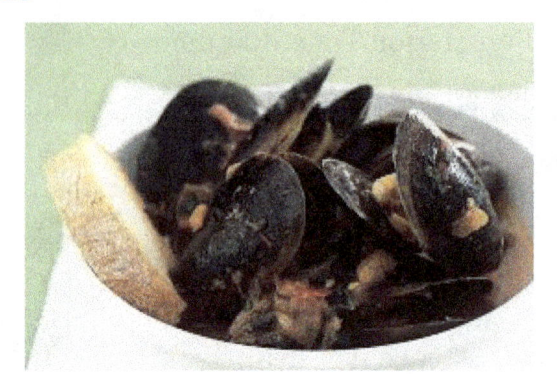

Nutrition:

- Calories 136
- Fat 4.7
- Fiber 0.6
- Carbs 7.5
- Protein 15.3

Mackerel Skillet with Greens

Preparation Time: 10 minutes

Cooking Time: 15 minutes

Servings: 4

Ingredients:

- 1 cup fresh spinach, chopped
- ½ cup endive, chopped
- 11 oz mackerel
- 1 tablespoon olive oil
- 1 teaspoon ground nutmeg
- ½ teaspoon salt
- ½ teaspoon turmeric
- ½ teaspoon chili flakes
- 3 tablespoons sour cream

Directions:

1. Pour olive oil in the skillet.
2. Add mackerel and sprinkle it with chili flakes, turmeric, and salt.
3. Roast fish for 2 minutes from each side.
4. Then add chopped endive, fresh spinach, and sour cream.
5. Mix up well and close the lid.
6. Simmer the meal for 10 minutes over the medium-low heat.

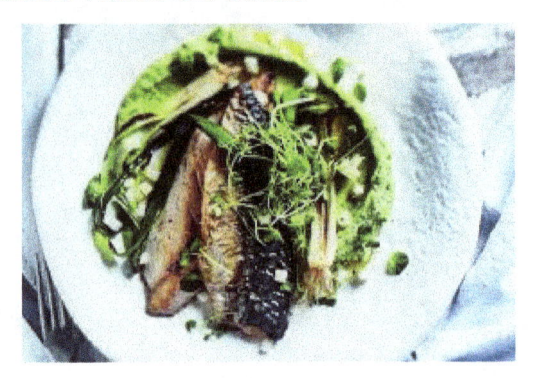

Nutrition:

- Calories 260
- Fat 19.5
- Fiber 0.5
- Carbs 1.3
- Protein 19.2

Shrimp Paella

Preparation time:5 minutes
Cooking time:10 minutes
Servings:2

Ingredients:

- 1 cup cooked brown rice
- 1 chopped red onion
- 1 tsp. paprika
- 1 chopped garlic clove
- 1 tbsp. olive oil
- 6 oz. frozen cooked shrimp
- 1 deseeded and sliced chili pepper
- 1 tbsp. oregano

Directions:

1. Heat the olive oil in a large pan on medium-high heat.
2. Add the onion and garlic and sauté for 2-3 minutes until soft.
3. Now add the shrimp and sauté for a further 5 minutes or until hot through.
4. Now add the herbs, spices, chili and rice with 1/2 cup boiling water.
5. Stir until everything is warm and the water has been absorbed.
6. Plate up and serve.

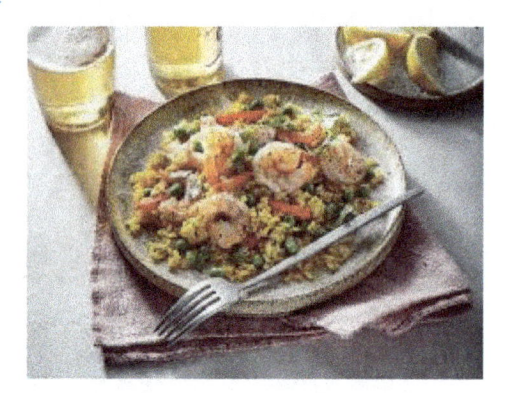

Nutrition:

- Calories 221
- Protein 17 g
- Carbs 31 g
- Fat 8 g
- Sodium (Na) 235 mg
- Potassium (K) 176 mg
- Phosphorus 189 mg

Fishen Papillote

Preparation Time: 15 minutes

Cooking Time: 20 minutes

Servings: 3

Ingredients:

- 10 oz snapper fillet
- 1 tablespoon fresh dill, chopped
- 1 white onion, peeled, sliced
- ½ teaspoon tarragon
- 1 tablespoon olive oil
- 1 teaspoon salt
- ½ teaspoon hot pepper
- 2 tablespoons sour cream

Directions:

1. Make the medium size packets from parchment and arrange them in the baking tray.
2. Cut the snapper fillet on 3 and sprinkle them with salt, tarragon, and hot pepper.
3. Put the fish fillets in the parchment packets.
4. Then top the fish with olive oil, sour cream sliced onion, and fresh dill.
5. Bake the fish for 20 minutes at 355F.

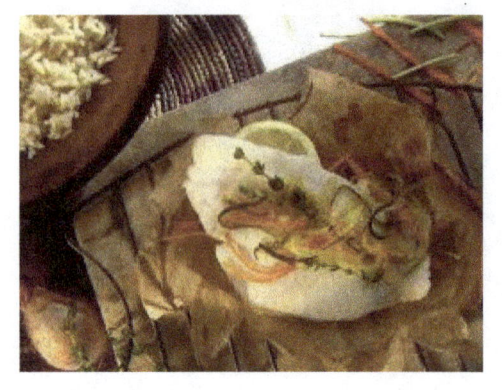

Nutrition:

- Calories 204
- Fat 8.2
- Fiber 1
- Carbs 4.6
- Protein 27.2

Herby Chicken Stew

Preparation time: 5 minutes
Cooking time: 40 minutes
Servings: 6

Ingredients:

- 10 oz. skinless and diced chicken breast
- ½ cup white rice
- ½ diced red onion
- 1 tsp. dried oregano
- 1 tsp. dried thyme
- 1 tsp. olive oil
- ½ cup diced eggplant
- Black pepper
- 1 cup water

Directions:

1. Soak vegetables in warm water prior to use if possible.
2. Heat an oven-proof pot over medium-high heat and add olive oil.
3. Add the diced chicken breast and brown in the pot for 5-6 minutes, stirring to brown each side.
4. Once the chicken is browned, lower the heat to medium and add the vegetables to the pot to sauté for 5-6 minutes - careful not to let the vegetables brown.
5. Add the water, herbs and pepper and bring to the boil.

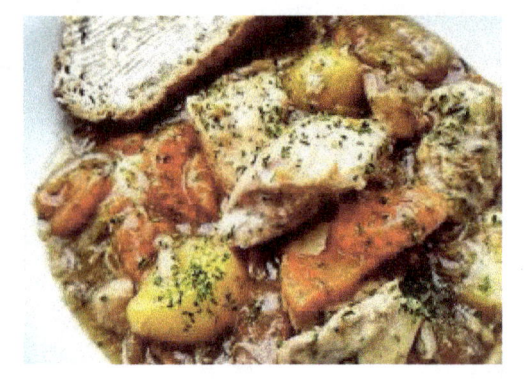

6. Reduce the heat and simmer (lid on) for 30-40 minutes or until chicken is thoroughly cooked through.
7. Meanwhile, prepare your rice by rinsing in cold water first and then adding to a pan of cold water and bringing to the boil over high heat.
8. Reduce the heat to medium and cook for 15 minutes.
9. Drain the rice and add back to the pan with the lid on to steam until the stew is ready.
10. Serve the stew on a bed of rice and enjoy!

Nutrition:

- Calories 143
- Protein 15 g
- Carbs 9 g
- Fat 5 g
- Sodium (Na) 12 mg
- Potassium (K) 20 mg
- Phosphorus 153 mg

Monk-Fish Curry

Preparation time: 5 minutes
Cooking time: 20 minutes
Servings: 2

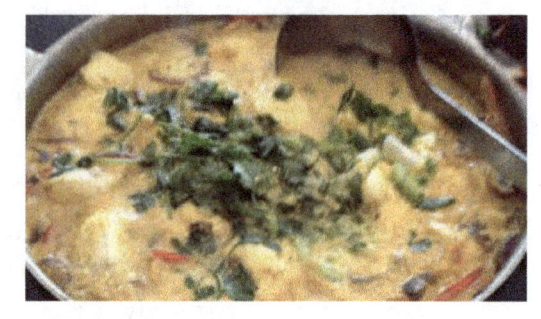

Ingredients:

- 1 garlic clove
- 3 finely chopped green onions
- 1 tsp. grated ginger
- 1 cup water.
- 2 tsps. Chopped fresh basil
- 1 cup cooked rice noodles
- 1 tbsp. coconut oil
- ½ sliced red chili
- 4 oz. Monk-fish fillet
- ½ finely sliced stick lemongrass
- 2 tbsps. chopped shallots

Directions:

1. Slice the Monkfish into bite-size pieces.
2. Using a pestle and mortar or food processor, crush the basil, garlic, ginger, chili and lemongrass to form a paste.
3. Heat the oil in a large wok or pan over medium-high heat and add the shallots.
4. Now add the water to the pan and bring to the boil.
5. Add the Monkfish, lower the heat and cover to simmer for 10 minutes or until cooked through.

6. Enjoy with rice noodles and scatter with green onions to serve.

Nutrition:

- Calories 249
- Protein 12 g
- Carbs 30 g
- Fat 10 g
- Sodium (Na) 32 mg
- Potassium (K) 398 mg
- Phosphorus 190 mg

Salmon Balls with Cream Cheese

Preparation Time: 15 minutes

Cooking Time: 15 minutes

Servings: 5

Ingredients:

- 1-pound salmon fillet
- 2 teaspoons cream cheese
- 3 tablespoons panko breadcrumbs
- ½ teaspoon salt
- 1 oz Parmesan, grated
- ½ teaspoon ground black pepper
- 1 teaspoon dried oregano
- 1 tablespoon sunflower oil

Directions:

1. Grind the salmon fillet and combine it together with cream cheese, panko breadcrumbs, salt, Parmesan, ground black pepper, and dried oregano.
2. Then make the small balls from the mixture and place them in the non-sticky tray.
3. Sprinkle the balls with sunflower oil and bake in the preheated to the 365F oven for 15 minutes. Flip the balls on another side after 10 minutes of cooking.

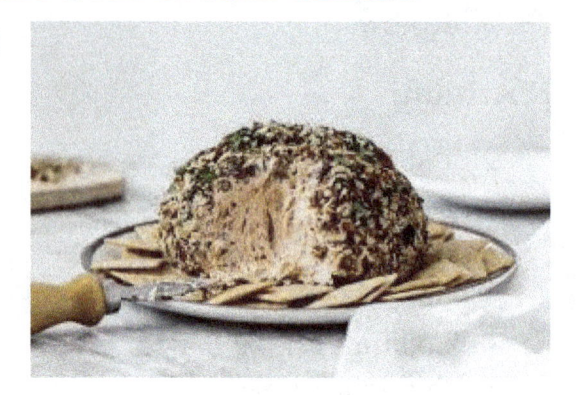

Nutrition:

- Calories 180
- Fat 10.2
- Fiber 0.5
- Carbs 2.8
- Protein 19.9

Poultry and Meat mains

Beef Brochettes

Preparation time:20 minutes
Cooking time:60 minutes
Servings:1

Ingredients:

- 1 ½ cups pineapple chunks
- 1 sliced large onion
- 2 lbs. thick steak
- 1 sliced medium bell pepper
- For the marinade:
- 1 bay leaf
- ¼ cup vegetable oil
- ½ cup lemon juice
- 2 crushed garlic cloves

Directions:

1. Cut beef cubes and place in a plastic bag
2. Combine marinade ingredients in small bowl
3. Mix and pour over beef cubes
4. Seal the bag and refrigerate for 3 to 5 hours
5. Divide ingredients: onion, beef cube, green pepper, pineapple
6. Grill about 9 minutes each side

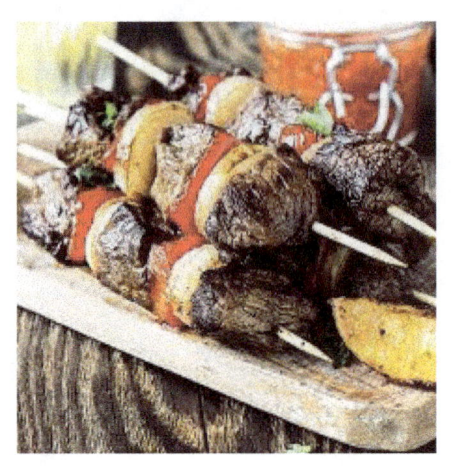

Nutrition:

- Calories 304
- Protein 35 g
- Fat 15 g
- Carbs 11 g
- Phosphorus 264 mg
- Potassium (K) 388 mg
- Sodium (Na) 70 mg

Meat Loaf

Preparation time: 20 minutes
Cooking time: 20 minutes
Servings: 1

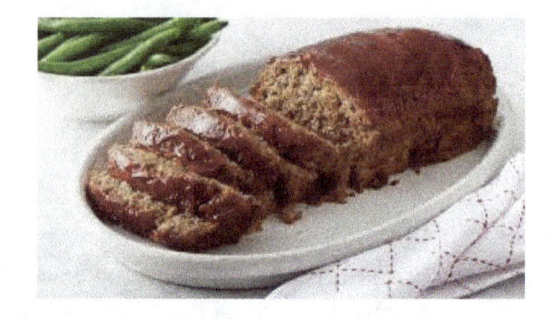

Ingredients:

- ½ tsp. ground sage
- 1 egg
- ¼ tsp. garlic powder
- 1 cup milk
- 1 tbsp. chopped parsley
- 4 soft bread slices
- ½ lb. lean ground pork
- ¼ tsp. pepper
- ¼ tsp. mustard
- 1 lb. lean ground beef
- ¼ cup onion

Directions:

1. Heat oven at 350 °F
2. Mix elements in a bowl
3. Place mixture in a shallow baking dish
4. Bake ½ hours or until done (At the end loaf should be crispy brown)

Nutrition:

- Calories 261
- Protein 27 g

- Fat 12 g
- Carbs 8 g
- Phosphorus 244 mg
- Potassium (K) 450 mg
- Sodium (Na) 180 mg

Chinese Beef Wraps

Preparation time: 10 minutes
Cooking time: 30 minutes
Servings: 2

Ingredients:

- 2 iceberg lettuce leaves
- ½ diced cucumber
- 1 tsp. canola oil
- 5 oz. lean ground beef
- 1 tsp. ground ginger
- 1 tbsp. chili flakes
- 1 minced garlic clove
- 1 tbsp. rice wine vinegar

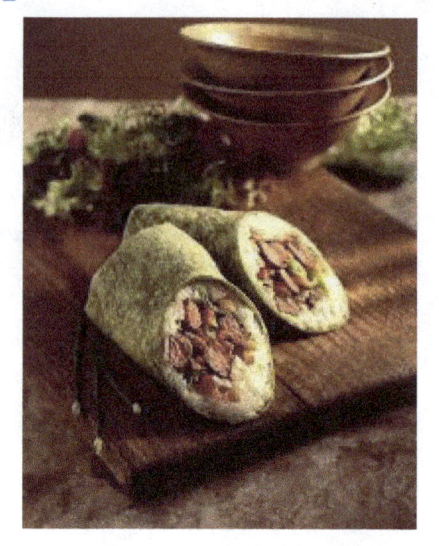

Directions:

1. Mix the ground meat with the garlic, rice wine vinegar, chili flakes and ginger in a bowl.
2. Heat oil in a skillet over medium heat.
3. Add the beef to the pan and cook for 20-25 minutes or until cooked through.
4. Serve beef mixture with diced cucumber in each lettuce wrap and fold.

Nutrition:

- Calories 156
- Fat 2g
- Carbs 4 g
- Phosphorus 1 mg
- Potassium (K) 78mg

- Sodium (Na) 54mg
- Protein 14g

Lamb with Zucchini & Couscous

Servings: 2

Preparation Time: 15 minutes

Cooking Time: 8 minutes

Ingredients:

- ¾ cup couscous
- ¾ cup boiling water
- ¼ cup fresh cilantro, chopped
- 1 tbsp olive oil
- 5-ounces lamb leg steak, cubed into ¾-inch size
- 1 medium zucchini, sliced thinly
- 1 medium red onion, cut into wedges
- 1 teaspoon ground cumin
- 1 teaspoon ground coriander
- ¼ teaspoon red pepper flakes, crushed
- Salt, to taste
- ¼ cup plain Greek yogurt
- 1 garlic herb, minced

Directions:

1. In a bowl, add couscous and boiling water and stir to combine,
2. Cover whilst aside approximately 5 minutes.
3. Add cilantro and with a fork, fluff completely.
4. Meanwhile in a substantial skillet, heat oil on high heat.
5. Add lamb and stir fry for about 2-3 minutes.

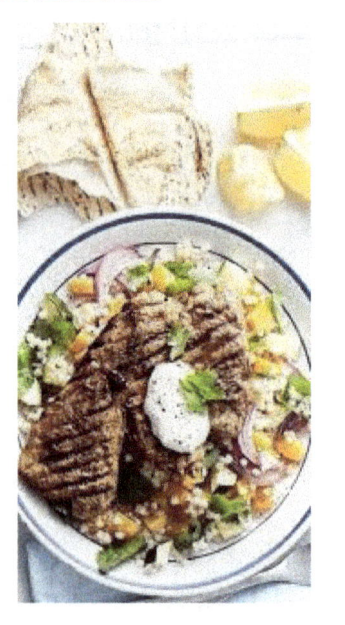

6. Add zucchini and onion and stir fry for about 2 minutes.
7. Stir in spices and stir fry for about 1 minute
8. Add couscous and stir fry approximately 2 minutes.
9. In a bowl, mix together yogurt and garlic.
10. Divide lamb mixture in serving plates evenly.
11. Serve using the topping of yogurt.

Nutrition:

- Calories 392
- Fat 5g
- Carbohydrates 2g
- Fiber 12g
- Protein 35g

Grilled Skirt Steak

Servings: 4

Preparation Time: 15 minutes

Cooking Time: 8-9 minutes

Ingredients:

- 2 teaspoons fresh ginger herb, grated finely
- 2 teaspoons fresh lime zest, grated finely
- ¼ cup coconut sugar
- 2 teaspoons fish sauce
- 2 tablespoons fresh lime juice
- ½ cup coconut milk
- 1-pound beef skirt steak, trimmed and cut into 4-inch slices lengthwise
- Salt, to taste

Directions:

1. In a sizable sealable bag, mix together all ingredients except steak and salt.
2. Add steak and coat with marinade generously.
3. Seal the bag and refrigerate to marinate for about 4-12 hours.
4. Preheat the grill to high heat. Grease the grill grate.
5. Remove steak from refrigerator and discard the marinade.
6. With a paper towel, dry the steak and sprinkle with salt evenly.

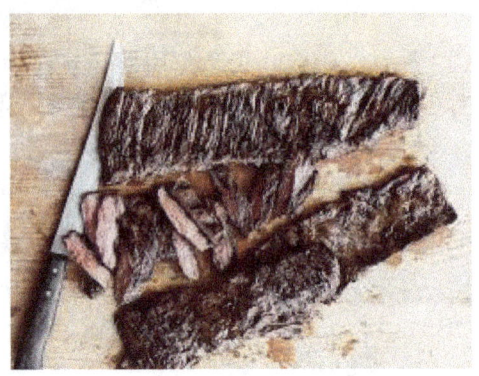

7. Cook the steak for approximately 3½ minutes.
8. Flip the medial side and cook for around 2½-5 minutes or till desired doneness.
9. Remove from grill pan and keep side for approximately 5 minutes before slicing.
10. With a clear, crisp knife cut into desired slices and serve.

Nutrition:

- Calories 465
- Fat 10g
- Carbohydrates 22g
- Fiber 0g
- Protein: 37g

Spiced Pork

One from the absolute delicious dish of spiced pork. Slow cooking helps you to infuse the spice flavors in pork very nicely.

Servings: 6

Preparation Time: fifteen minutes

Cooking Time: 1 hour 52 minutes

Ingredients:

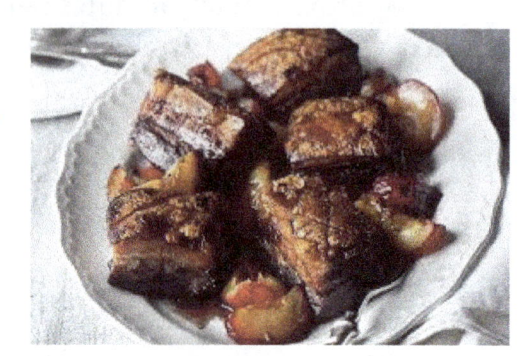

- 1 (2-inch) piece fresh ginger, chopped
- 5-10 garlic cloves, chopped
- 1 teaspoon ground cumin
- ½ teaspoon ground turmeric
- 1 tablespoon hot paprika
- 1 tablespoon red pepper flakes
- Salt, to taste
- 2 tablespoons cider vinegar
- 2-pounds pork shoulder, trimmed and cubed into 1½-inch size
- 2 cups domestic hot water, divided
- 1 (1-inch wide) ball tamarind pulp
- ¼ cup olive oil
- 1 teaspoon black mustard seeds, crushed
- 4 green cardamoms
- 5 whole cloves
- 1 (3-inch) cinnamon stick
- 1 cup onion, chopped finely

- 1 large red bell pepper, seeded and chopped

Directions:

1. In a food processor, add ginger, garlic, cumin, turmeric, paprika, red pepper flakes, salt and cider vinegar and pulse till smooth.
2. Transfer the amalgamation into a large bowl.
3. Add pork and coat with mixture generously.
4. Keep aside, covered for around an hour at room temperature.
5. In a bowl, add 1 cup of warm water and tamarind and make aside till water becomes cool.
6. With the hands, crush the tamarind to extract the pulp.
7. Add remaining cup of hot water and mix till well combined.
8. Through a fine sieve, strain the tamarind juice inside a bowl.
9. In a sizable skillet, heat oil on medium-high heat.
10. Add mustard seeds, green cardamoms, cloves and cinnamon stick and sauté for about 4 minutes.
11. Add onion and sauté for approximately 5 minutes.
12. Add pork and stir fry for approximately 6 minutes.
13. Stir in tamarind juice and convey with a boil.
14. Reduce the heat to medium-low and simmer 1½ hours.
15. Stir in bell pepper and cook for about 7 minutes.

Nutrition:

- Calories 435
- Fat 16g
- Carbohydrates 27g

- Fiber 3g
- Protein 39g

Spicy Lamb Curry

Servings: 6-8

Preparation Time: 15 minutes

Cooking Time: 2 hours 15 minutes

Ingredients:

- For Spice Mixture:
    - 4 teaspoons ground coriander
    - 4 teaspoons ground coriander
    - 4 teaspoons ground cumin
    - ¾ teaspoon ground ginger
    - 2 teaspoons ground cinnamon
    - ½ teaspoon ground cloves
    - ½ teaspoon ground cardamom
    - 2 tablespoons sweet paprika
    - ½ tablespoon cayenne pepper
    - 2 teaspoons chili powder
    - 2 teaspoons salt
- For Curry:
    - 1 tablespoon coconut oil
    - 2 pounds boneless lamb, trimmed and cubed into 1-inch size
    - Salt and freshly ground black pepper, to taste
    - 2 cups onions, chopped
    - 1¼ cups water
    - 1 cup coconut milk

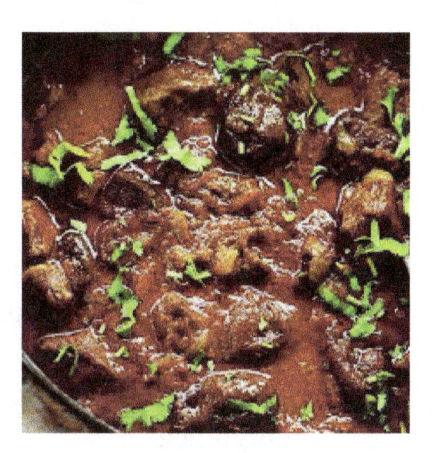

Directions:

1. For spice mixture in a bowl, mix together all spices. Keep aside.
2. Season the lamb with salt and black pepper.
3. In a large Dutch oven, heat oil on medium-high heat.
4. Add lamb and stir fry for around 5 minutes.
5. Add onion and cook approximately 4-5 minutes.
6. Stir in spice mixture and cook approximately 1 minute.
7. Add water and coconut milk and provide to some boil on high heat.
8. Reduce the heat to low and simmer, covered for approximately 1-120 minutes or till desired doneness of lamb.
9. Uncover and simmer for approximately 3-4 minutes.
10. Serve hot.

Nutrition:

- Calories 466
- Fat 10g
- Carbohydrates 23g
- Fiber 9g
- Protein 36g

Roast Beef

Preparation time: 25 minutes
Cooking time: 55 minutes,
Serves: 3

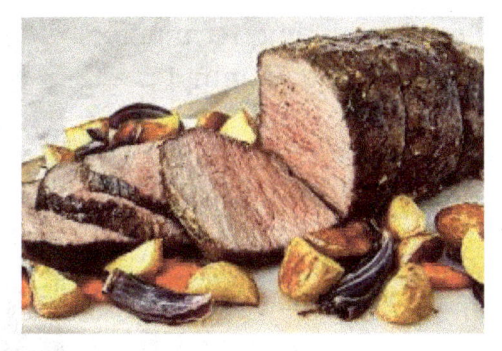

Ingredients:

- Quality rump or sirloin tip roast

Directions:

1. Place in roasting pan o n a shallow rack
2. Season with pepper and herbs
3. Insert meat thermometer in the center or thickest part of the roast
4. Roast to the desired degree of doneness
5. After removing from over for about 15 minutes let it chill
6. In the end the roast should be moister than well done.

Nutrition:

- Calories 158
- Protein 24 g
- Fat 6 g
- Carbs 0 g
- Phosphorus 206 mg
- Potassium (K) 328 mg
- Sodium (Na) 55 mg

Spiced Lamb Burgers

Preparation time:10 minutes
Cooking time:20 minutes
Servings:2

Ingredients:

- 1 tbsp. extra virgin olive oil
- 1 tsp. cumin
- ½ finely diced red onion 1 minced garlic clove
- 1 tsp. harissa spices
- 1 cup arugula
- 1 juiced lemon
- 6 oz. lean ground lamb
- 1 tbsp. parsley
- ½ cup low-fat plain yogurt

Directions:

1. Preheat the broiler on a medium to high heat.
2. Mix together the ground lamb, red onion, parsley, Harissa spices and olive oil until combined.
3. Shape 1-inch thick patties using wet hands.
4. Add the patties to a baking tray and place under the broiler for 7-8 minutes on each side or until thoroughly cooked through.
5. Mix the yogurt, lemon juice and cumin and serve over the lamb burgers with a side salad of arugula.

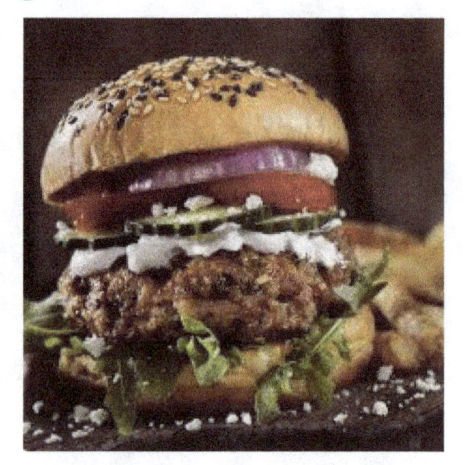

Nutrition:

- Calories 306
- Fat 20g
- Carbs 10g
- Phosphorus 269mg
- Potassium (K) 492mg
- Sodium (Na) 86mg
- Protein 23g

Lemon & Herb Chicken Wraps

Preparation time: 5 minutes
Cooking time: 30 minutes
Servings: 4

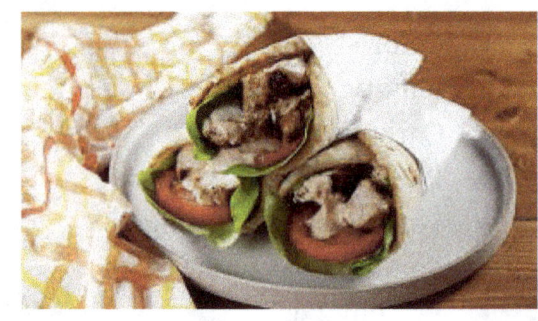

Ingredients:

- 4 oz. skinless and sliced chicken breasts
- ½ sliced red bell pepper
- 1 lemon
- 4 large iceberg lettuce leaves
- 1 tbsp. olive oil
- 2 tbsps. Finely chopped fresh cilantro
- ¼ tsp. black pepper

Directions:

1. Preheat the oven to 375°F/Gas Mark 5.
2. Mix the oil, juice of ½ lemon, cilantro and black pepper.
3. Marinate the chicken in the oil marinade, cover and leave in the fridge for as long as possible.
4. Wrap the chicken in parchment paper, drizzling over the remaining marinade.
5. Place in the oven in an oven dish for 25-30 minutes or until chicken is thoroughly cooked through and white inside.
6. Divide the sliced bell pepper and layer onto each lettuce leaf.
7. Divide the chicken onto each lettuce leaf and squeeze over the remaining lemon juice to taste.

8. Season with a little extra black pepper if desired.
9. Wrap and enjoy!

Nutrition:

- Calories 200
- Protein 9 g
- Carbs 5 g
- Fat 13 g
- Sodium (Na) 25 mg
- Potassium (K) 125 mg
- Phosphorus 81 mg

Vegetables mains

Delicious Vegetarian Lasagne

Preparation time:10 minutes
Cooking time:1 hour

Servings:4

Ingredients:

- 1 tsp. basil
- 1 tbsp. olive oil
- ½ sliced red pepper
- 3 lasagna sheets
- ½ diced red onion
- ¼ tsp. black pepper
- 1 cup rice milk
- 1 minced garlic clove
- 1 cup sliced eggplant
- ½ sliced zucchini
- ½ pack soft tofu
- 1 tsp. oregano

Directions:

1. Preheat oven to 325°F/Gas Mark 3.
2. Slice zucchini, eggplant and pepper into vertical strips.
3. Add the rice milk and tofu to a food processor and blitz until smooth. Set aside.
4. Heat the oil in a skillet over medium heat and add the onions and garlic for 3-4 minutes or until soft.

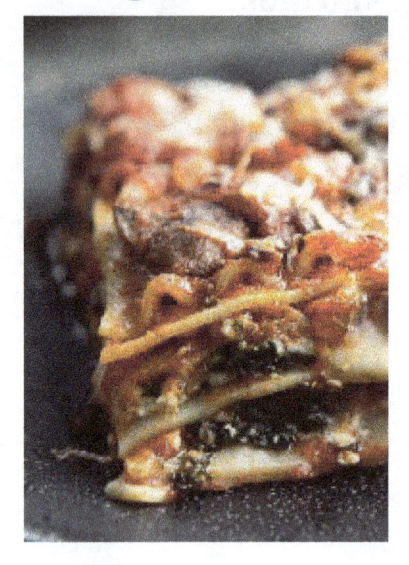

5. Sprinkle in the herbs and pepper and allow to stir through for 5-6 minutes until hot.
6. Into a lasagne or suitable oven dish, layer 1 lasagna sheet, then 1/3 the eggplant, followed by 1/3 zucchini, then 1/3 pepper before pouring over 1/3 of tofu white sauce.
7. Repeat for the next 2 layers, finishing with the white sauce.
8. Add to the oven for 40-50 minutes or until veg is soft and can easily be sliced into servings.

Nutrition:

- Calories 235
- Protein 5 g
- Carbs 10g
- Fat 9 g
- Sodium (Na) 35 mg
- Potassium (K) 129 mg
- Phosphorus 66 mg

Mixed Pepper Paella

Preparation time: 10 minutes
Cooking time: 35-40 minutes
Servings: 2

Ingredients:

- 1 tbsp. extra virgin olive oil
- ½ chopped red onion
- 1 lemon
- ½ chopped yellow bell pepper
- 1 cup homemade chicken broth
- ½ chopped zucchini
- 1 tsp. dried oregano
- ½ chopped red bell pepper
- 1 tsp. dried parsley
- 1 cup brown rice
- 1 tsp. paprika

Directions:

1. Add the rice to a pot of cold water and cook for 15 minutes.
2. Drain the water, cover the pan and leave to one side.
3. Heat the oil in a skillet over medium-high heat.
4. Add the bell peppers, onion and zucchini, sautéing for 5 minutes.
5. To the pan, add the rice, herbs, spices and juice of the lemon along with the chicken broth.

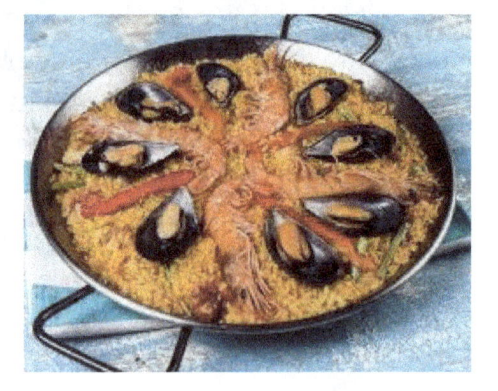

6. Cover and turn the heat right down and allow to simmer for 15-20 minutes.
7. Serve hot.

Nutrition:

- Calories 210
- Protein 4 g
- Carbs 33 g
- Fat 7 g
- Sodium (Na) 20 mg
- Potassium (K) 33 mg
- Phosphorus 156 mg

Lentil Vegan Soup

Servings: 5

Calories: 364 calories per serving

Preparation Time: 10 minutes

Cooking Time: 50 minutes

Ingredients:

- Olive oil - 2 tablespoons
- Onion (diced) - 1
- Garlic (minced) - 2 cloves
- Carrot (diced) - 1
- Potatoes (diced) - 2
- Tomato (diced) - 1 can (15 ounces)
- Dried lentil - 2 cups
- Vegetable broth - 8 cups
- Bay leaf - 1
- Cumin - ½ teaspoon
- Salt – as per taste
- Pepper – as per taste

Directions:

1. Start by taking a large pot and add in 2 tablespoons of olive oil. Place the pot over medium flame.
2. Once the oil heats through, toss in the onions and cook for 5 minutes.
3. Add in the garlic and cook for another 2 minutes.
4. Now toss in the diced potatoes and carrots. Sauté for about 3 minutes.

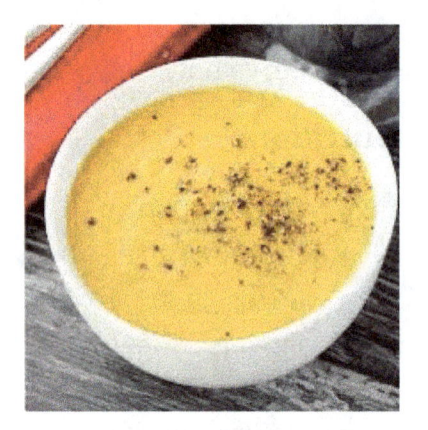

5. Add the remaining ingredients like vegetable broth, tomatoes, lentils, cumin and bay leaf.
6. Once it comes to a boil, reduce the flame to low and cook for about 40 minutes.
7. Remove the bay leaf and season with pepper and salt.
8. Transfer into a serving bowl. Serve hot!

Nutrition:

- Fat 7 g
- Carbohydrates 58 g
- Protein 19 g

Thai Tofu Broth

Preparation time:5 minutes
Cooking time:15 minutes
Servings:4

Ingredients:

- 1 cup rice noodles
- ½ sliced onion
- 6 oz. drained, pressed and cubed tofu
- ¼ cup sliced scallions
- ½ cup water
- ½ cup canned water chestnuts
- ½ cup rice milk
- 1 tbsp. lime juice
- 1 tbsp. coconut oil
- ½ finely sliced chili
- 1 cup snow peas

Directions:

1. Heat the oil in a wok on a high heat and then sauté the tofu until brown on each side.
2. Add the onion and sauté for 2-3 minutes.
3. Add the rice milk and water to the wok until bubbling.
4. Lower to medium heat and add the noodles, chili and water chestnuts.
5. Allow to simmer for 10-15 minutes and then add the sugar snap peas for 5 minutes.
6. Serve with a sprinkle of scallions.

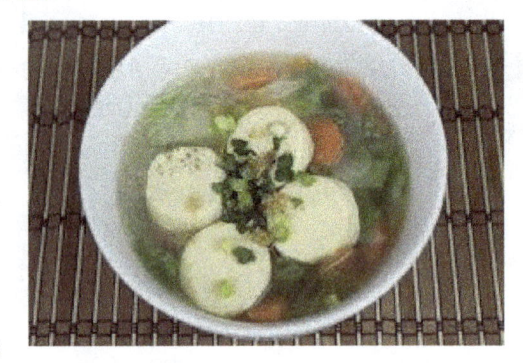

Nutrition:

- Calories 304
- Protein 9 g
- Carbs 38 g
- Fat 13 g
- Sodium (Na) 36 mg
- Potassium (K) 114 mg
- Phosphorus 101 mg

Chinese Tempeh Stir Fry

Preparation time: 5 minutes
Cooking time: 15 minutes
Servings: 2

Ingredients:

- 2 oz. sliced tempeh
- 1 cup cooked brown rice
- 1 minced garlic clove
- ½ cup green onions
- 1 tsp. minced fresh ginger
- 1 tbsp. coconut oil
- ½ cup corn

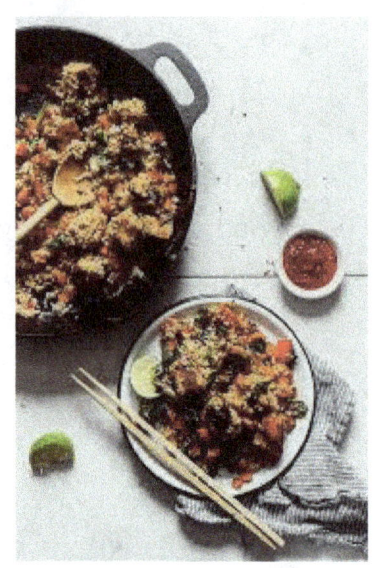

Directions:

1. Heat the oil in a skillet or wok on a high heat and add the garlic and ginger.
2. Sauté for 1 minute.
3. Now add the tempeh and cook for 5-6 minutes before adding the corn for a further 10 minutes.
4. Now add the green onions and serve over brown rice.

Nutrition:

- Calories 304
- Protein 10 g
- Carbs 35 g
- Fat 4 g
- Sodium (Na) 91 mg
- Potassium (K) 121 mg
- Phosphorus 222 mg

Minted Zucchini Noodles

Preparation time: 5 minutes
Cooking time: 10 minutes
Servings: 2

Ingredients:

- ¼ deseeded and chopped red chili
- 2 tbsps. Extra virgin olive oil
- ½ juiced lemon
- 4 peeled and sliced zucchinis
- ½ cup chopped fresh mint
- 1 tsp. black pepper
- ½ cup arugula

Directions:

1. Whisk the mint, pepper, chili and olive oil to make a dressing.
2. Meanwhile, heat a pan of water on a high heat and bring to the boil.
3. Add the zucchini noodles and turn the heat down to simmer for 3-4 minutes.
4. Remove from the heat and place in a bowl of cold water immediately.
5. Toss the noodles in the dressing.
6. Mix the arugula with the lemon juice to serve on the top.
7. Enjoy!

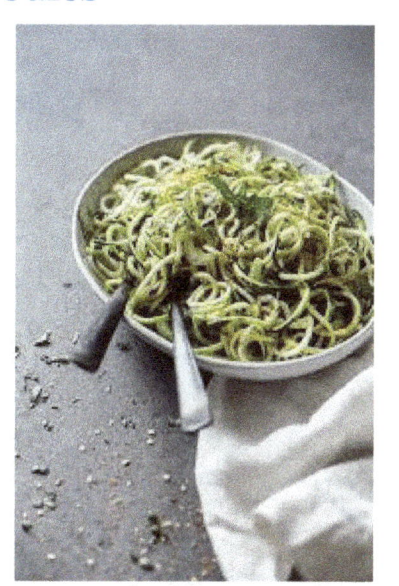

Nutrition:

- Calories 148
- Protein 2 g
- Carbs 4 g
- Fat 13 g
- Sodium (Na) 7 mg
- Potassium (K) 422 mg
- Phosphorus 256 mg

Vegan Alfredo Fettuccine Pasta

Servings: 2

Calories: 844 calories per serving

Preparation Time: 15 minutes

Cooking Time: 15 minutes

Ingredients:

- White potatoes - 2 medium
- White onion - ¼
- Italian seasoning - 1 tablespoon
- Lemon juice - 1 teaspoon
- Garlic - 2 cloves
- Salt - 1 teaspoon
- Fettuccine pasta - 12 ounces
- Raw cashew - ½ cup

Directions:

1. Start by placing a pot on high flame and boiling 4 cups of water.
2. Peel the potatoes and cut them into small cubes. Cut the onion into cubes as well.
3. Add the potatoes and onions to the boiling water and cook for about 10 minutes.
4. Remove the onions and potatoes. Keep aside. Save the water.
5. Take another pot and fill it with water. Season generously with salt.

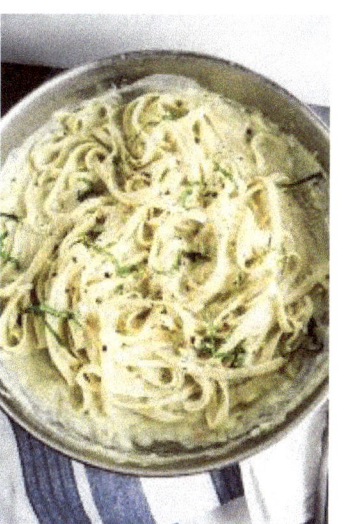

6. Toss in the fettuccine pasta and cook as per package instructions.
7. Take a blender and add in the raw cashews, veggies, nutritional yeast, truffle oil, lemon juice and 1 cup of saved water. Blend into a smooth puree.
8. Add in the garlic and salt.
9. Drain the cooked pasta using a colander. Transfer into a mixing bowl.
10. Pour the prepared sauce on top of the cooked fettuccine pasta. Serve.
11. Nutritional yeast (optional) - 1 teaspoon
12. Truffle oil (optional) - ¼ teaspoon

Nutrition:

- Fat 13 g
- Carbohydrates 152 g
- Protein 28 g